THE ALKALINE DIET COOKBOOK

A beginner guide to The Alkaline A Culinary Journey to Balance and Wellness

Dr Philip Ortner

Table of Contents

CHAPTER 1

Introduction to Alkaline Living

Welcome to the transformative world of alkaline living, where the journey begins towards a healthier, more balanced you. In this chapter, we'll delve into the fundamentals of the alkaline diet, unraveling its principles, and understanding the incredible benefits that come with maintaining a balanced pH level in the body. We'll also take a stroll through the aisles of alkaline-forming and acidic-forming foods, guiding you towards informed choices that will set the stage for a vibrant, alkaline life.

Explanation of the Alkaline Diet and Its Principles

At its core, the alkaline diet is centered around the concept of balance. Just like a tightrope walker maintains equilibrium, our bodies strive to achieve a delicate balance too, and the alkaline diet supports this equilibrium by promoting foods that help maintain an optimal pH level. But what does pH mean?

In simple terms, pH is a scale that measures how acidic or alkaline a substance is. The scale ranges from 0 to 14, where 0 is highly acidic, 14 is highly alkaline, and 7 is neutral. The human body operates best in a slightly alkaline environment, ideally around 7.35 to 7.45 pH. When we consume foods, they either leave an acidic or alkaline residue in our bodies. The alkaline diet encourages us to focus on foods that leave an alkaline residue, promoting this slightly alkaline state and supporting overall well-being.

The principles of the alkaline diet revolve around consuming a variety of alkaline-forming foods such as fruits, vegetables, nuts, and seeds, while minimizing the intake of acidic-forming foods like processed foods, dairy, and certain grains. By adopting this approach, we provide our bodies with the tools needed to maintain a more alkaline pH, reducing the risk of inflammation, supporting immune function, and contributing to long-term health.

Benefits of Maintaining a Balanced pH Level

Why is maintaining a balanced pH level so crucial for our health? Think of your body as a well-coordinated orchestra. Each instrument (organ) plays a specific role, and for the symphony to sound harmonious, the pH levels need to be in tune.

When our body becomes too acidic, it creates an environment that can lead to inflammation, weakened immune function, and increased vulnerability to diseases. On the other hand, maintaining a slightly alkaline pH supports cellular function, aids in nutrient absorption, and provides an environment where the body can thrive.

An alkaline environment is like a shield, protecting us from the stresses of modern life, pollution, and the consumption of processed foods. It's not just about feeling good; it's about empowering our body's natural defense mechanisms to function optimally.

Overview of Alkaline-Forming and Acidic-Forming Foods

Now, let's explore the colorful palette of foods that either contribute to an alkaline or acidic environment within our bodies.

Alkaline-Forming Foods:

- **Fruits and Vegetables:** Packed with vitamins, minerals, and antioxidants, these are the superheroes of the alkaline diet. Examples include leafy greens, berries, citrus fruits, and cruciferous vegetables like broccoli and kale.

- **Nuts and Seeds:** Almonds, chia seeds, and flaxseeds are excellent choices. They not only add a delightful crunch to your meals but also contribute to alkalinity.

- **Healthy Oils:** Olive oil and coconut oil fall into this category, providing healthy fats that support overall well-being.

- **Alkaline Water:** Staying hydrated is key, and alkaline water can be a refreshing choice that aligns with the principles of the diet.

Acidic-Forming Foods:

- **Processed Foods:** Fast food, sugary snacks, and heavily processed items often lead to acidity in the body.

- **Dairy:** While dairy products are rich in calcium, they can contribute to acidity. Consider alternative options like almond or coconut milk.

- **Meat:** While some forms of meat can be part of a balanced diet, excessive consumption, especially of red and processed meats, can tip the pH balance toward acidity.

- **Caffeine and Alcohol:** While enjoyable in moderation, excessive coffee and alcohol intake can have acidic effects.

Understanding the distinction between these two groups empowers you to make mindful choices when planning your meals, ensuring that you create a menu that supports your journey towards a more alkaline lifestyle.

CHAPTER 2

The Science Behind Alkalinity

Welcome to the heart of understanding alkalinity – the science that underpins the transformative power of the alkaline diet. In this chapter, we'll embark on a journey into the intricacies of the pH scale, demystifying its relevance to our health. We'll explore how the foods we consume influence the delicate balance within, paving the way for a more harmonious internal environment. Additionally, we'll shine a light on the consequences of acidity, unraveling its impact on our overall well-being in terms that resonate with our daily lives.

In-depth Exploration of the pH Scale and Its Relevance to Health

Imagine the pH scale as a thermometer for your body's internal climate. This scale ranges from 0 to 14, with 7 being neutral, lower numbers indicating acidity, and higher numbers indicating alkalinity. Our bodies, being the incredible biological marvels they are, operate optimally at a slightly alkaline pH, specifically around 7.35 to 7.45.

To put it in perspective, think of your body as a swimming pool. You want the water to be just right – not too acidic, not too alkaline. If it's too acidic, it can irritate your skin and eyes. If it's too alkaline, it can lead to cloudy water. Similarly, our bodies function best when the internal environment is slightly alkaline. This sets the stage for optimal cellular function, efficient nutrient absorption, and a balanced immune system.

Now, how do the foods we eat impact this internal pH? Different foods leave behind different residues after digestion. Alkaline-forming foods, rich in essential nutrients and antioxidants, leave an alkaline residue, contributing to the pool of health-promoting elements in our bodies. On the other hand, acidic-forming foods, often processed and lacking in nutritional density, contribute to an acidic residue, tipping the balance towards an environment that may foster inflammation and compromise well-being.

How Alkaline Foods Contribute to a More Balanced Internal Environment

Let's envision your body as a bustling city. The citizens of this city are the cells, and just like any thriving community, they need a clean and balanced environment to function optimally. Alkaline-forming foods act as the city planners, ensuring that the streets are clean, the air is fresh, and the infrastructure is robust.

These foods, primarily fruits, vegetables, nuts, and seeds, bring with them an arsenal of vitamins, minerals, and antioxidants. They are like the architects of a well-designed cityscape, constructing strong buildings (cells) and providing the necessary resources for a flourishing community. The alkaline residue they leave behind acts as a foundation for a resilient and balanced internal environment.

On the contrary, imagine acidic-forming foods as pollutants in our city. They clog the streets, pollute the air, and put a strain on the city's resources. Similarly, processed foods, excessive meat consumption, and sugary treats, common culprits of acidity, burden our bodies with inflammatory residues. Over time, this can lead to cellular stress, compromise the immune system, and create an environment that is less conducive to overall health.

Impact of Acidity on Overall Well-being

Now, let's discuss the consequences of living in an overly acidic environment. Picture a garden overwhelmed by weeds; the vibrant, life-sustaining plants struggle to thrive. Similarly, when our bodies become too acidic, the optimal conditions for health diminish, and the consequences are far-reaching.

1. **Inflammation:** Acidity is like fuel to the fire of inflammation. Chronic inflammation is linked to various health issues, including arthritis,

cardiovascular diseases, and even certain cancers. Alkaline foods act as firefighters, helping to dampen the flames of inflammation and restore balance.

2. **Weakened Immune Function:** The immune system, our body's defense force, operates more efficiently in an alkaline environment. When the body becomes too acidic, the immune system may become compromised, making us more susceptible to infections and illnesses.

3. **Fatigue and Low Energy:** Picture your body as an engine. In an alkaline environment, it runs smoothly and efficiently. In an acidic environment, it sputters and struggles. This can manifest as fatigue, low energy levels, and a general sense of sluggishness.

4. **Digestive Issues:** An overly acidic environment can disrupt the delicate balance of the digestive system, leading to issues like acid reflux, indigestion, and an increased risk of developing conditions such as irritable bowel syndrome (IBS).

Understanding the impact of acidity on our bodies is a crucial step toward embracing the alkaline lifestyle. It's not just about numbers on a pH scale; it's about cultivating an internal environment that fosters vitality, resilience, and overall well-being.

CHAPTER 3

Setting Up Your Alkaline Kitchen

Welcome to the heart of your alkaline journey—the kitchen. This chapter is your blueprint for transforming your cooking space into a haven of health and balance. We'll dive into the essential ingredients that will stock your alkaline pantry, explore the kitchen tools and equipment that will make alkaline cooking a breeze, and unravel practical tips for meal planning and preparation. Get ready to turn your kitchen into a powerhouse of alkaline delight.

Essential Ingredients for an Alkaline Pantry

Imagine your pantry as a treasure trove of health, packed with ingredients that support your body's journey towards balance. Let's explore the key players in your alkaline pantry:

1. **Fresh Fruits and Vegetables:** The backbone of the alkaline diet. Load up on colorful fruits and a variety of vegetables. Leafy greens like kale and spinach, vibrant bell peppers, and citrus fruits are fantastic choices.
2. **Nuts and Seeds:** Almonds, walnuts, chia seeds, and flaxseeds are not only great for snacking but also add a delightful crunch and a nutritional boost to your meals.
3. **Whole Grains:** Opt for alkaline grains like quinoa, millet, and amaranth. These grains are not only nutritious but also versatile, forming the base for many alkaline meals.
4. **Healthy Oils:** Olive oil and coconut oil are your go-to choices. They not only add rich flavors to your dishes but also contribute to the alkaline environment you're aiming for.

5. **Herbs and Spices:** Flavor is key, and you'll be delighted by the array of alkaline-friendly herbs and spices. Turmeric, ginger, cilantro, and basil can elevate your dishes while providing additional health benefits.

6. **Alkaline Water:** Staying hydrated is fundamental. Consider investing in a water filter to ensure that your hydration source aligns with the principles of the alkaline diet.

7. **Plant-Based Proteins:** Legumes like chickpeas, lentils, and black beans, along with tofu and tempeh, offer excellent sources of protein without the acidic load associated with some animal proteins.

8. **Alkaline-Friendly Sweeteners:** Stevia and agave nectar are sweet alternatives that won't tip the pH balance.

Building an alkaline pantry is about filling your shelves with whole, unprocessed foods that are rich in nutrients and contribute to the alkaline environment your body craves.

Kitchen Tools and Equipment for Alkaline Cooking

Now that your pantry is stocked, let's explore the tools that will turn your ingredients into culinary delights:

1. **High-Quality Blender:** Perfect for creating alkaline smoothies, soups, and sauces. Invest in a blender that can handle a variety of textures, from leafy greens to nuts.
2. **Juicer:** Freshly squeezed alkaline juices can be a refreshing addition to your routine. Look for a juicer that retains maximum nutrients from your fruits and vegetables.
3. **Steamer Basket:** A simple and effective way to cook vegetables while preserving their nutritional content. Steaming is an alkaline-friendly cooking method.

4. **Non-Stick Pans:** Opt for non-stick pans to reduce the need for excessive oils when cooking. Stainless steel or ceramic-coated pans are excellent choices.

5. **Food Processor:** From chopping nuts to creating alkaline dips and spreads, a food processor is a versatile tool that will save you time in the kitchen.

6. **Alkaline Water Filter:** Ensure that the water you use in your recipes aligns with the alkaline principles. A water filter can help remove impurities.

7. **Sharp Knives:** A set of sharp knives will make chopping and slicing fruits and vegetables a breeze. Precision in cutting helps retain the nutritional value of your ingredients.

8. **Mason Jars and Glass Containers:** Perfect for storing alkaline-rich salads, soups, and leftovers. Glass containers are preferable to avoid any leaching from plastic.

Tips for Meal Planning and Preparation:

Meal planning is your secret weapon in maintaining an alkaline lifestyle. Here are some tips to make it a seamless part of your routine:

1. **Batch Cooking:** Dedicate a day to batch cook staples like quinoa, beans, and roasted vegetables. This makes assembling meals during the week quick and easy.
2. **Colorful Plate Rule:** Aim to have a variety of colors on your plate. The vibrant pigments in fruits and vegetables often indicate a rich array of nutrients.
3. **Plan Your Protein:** Ensure that each meal includes a good source of plant-based protein. This can be beans, lentils, tofu, or a combination of these.
4. **Hydration Habits:** Sip on alkaline water throughout the day. Consider infusing it with slices of lemon or cucumber for added flavor.

5. **Snack Smart:** Keep alkaline snacks, such as a handful of almonds or sliced veggies with hummus, readily available to curb cravings.

6. **Experiment with Herbs and Spices:** Use herbs and spices liberally to add flavor without relying on acidic condiments.

7. **Mindful Eating:** Take time to savor your meals. Eating slowly and mindfully can enhance digestion and nutrient absorption.

By setting up your kitchen with these essentials and incorporating these practical tips into your routine, you're not just preparing meals; you're cultivating a lifestyle that supports your journey towards balance and well-being.

CHAPTER 4

Breakfasts for Energy and Vitality

Welcome to the sunshine of your alkaline day — breakfast! This chapter is your morning muse, guiding you through alkaline breakfast recipes that will kickstart your day with energy and vitality. From refreshing smoothies to comforting porridges and nourishing breakfast bowls, we'll explore delicious ways to embrace the alkaline lifestyle. Additionally, we'll uncover the importance of alkaline morning rituals, setting the tone for a day filled with balance and well-being.

Alkaline Breakfast Recipes to Kickstart Your Day

Breakfast is your body's wake-up call, and an alkaline breakfast ensures that it rises and shines with vitality. Let's explore some delightful recipes that not only taste great but also align with the principles of the alkaline diet:

1. **Green Smoothie Bliss:**
   - Ingredients: Spinach, kale, cucumber, celery, green apple, lemon, and a handful of almonds.
   - Method: Blend all the ingredients with alkaline water for a refreshing and nutrient-packed green smoothie. The greens provide essential vitamins, while almonds add a protein boost.
2. **Quinoa Breakfast Bowl:**
   - Ingredients: Cooked quinoa, mixed berries, sliced banana, and a drizzle of agave nectar.
   - Method: Combine the cooked quinoa with the fruits and top it off with a touch of agave nectar. This bowl is a satisfying blend of alkaline grains and antioxidant-rich berries.
3. **Chia Seed Pudding:**

- o Ingredients: Chia seeds, almond milk, vanilla extract, and a topping of sliced kiwi and strawberries.
- o Method: Mix chia seeds with almond milk and vanilla extract, then refrigerate overnight. In the morning, top it with fresh fruit for a delightful chia seed pudding that's rich in omega-3 fatty acids.

4. **Alkaline Oatmeal:**
- o Ingredients: Rolled oats, almond milk, sliced almonds, and diced pear.
- o Method: Cook the rolled oats with almond milk, top it with sliced almonds, and add diced pear for a heartwarming and alkaline-rich oatmeal.

5. **Avocado Toast with Tomato Salsa:**
- o Ingredients: Whole-grain toast, mashed avocado, and a salsa of diced tomatoes, red onion, cilantro, and lime juice.
- o Method: Spread mashed avocado on whole-grain toast and top it with a zesty tomato

salsa. This breakfast is a perfect combination of healthy fats and alkaline vegetables.

Smoothies, Porridges, and Breakfast Bowls

These breakfast options aren't just about fueling your body; they're a celebration of flavors and textures that make mornings something to look forward to.

1. **Smoothies:**
   - Smoothies are like a nutritional symphony in a glass. They blend the goodness of fruits, vegetables, and nuts into a harmonious concoction that's both refreshing and energizing. The fiber from greens and fruits supports digestion, while nuts provide a satiating protein boost.

2. **Porridges:**
   - A warm bowl of porridge is the epitome of comfort, and when it's made with alkaline

grains like quinoa or oats, it becomes a nutritional powerhouse. Add fruits, nuts, and a touch of natural sweetener for a breakfast that warms your body and nourishes your soul.

3. **Breakfast Bowls:**

   o Breakfast bowls are a canvas for creativity. Whether it's a quinoa bowl with vibrant berries or a chia seed pudding adorned with tropical fruits, these bowls are a feast for the eyes and the body. The combination of textures and flavors makes them a delightful way to start your day.

The Importance of Alkaline Morning Rituals

Your morning routine sets the tone for the entire day. Incorporating alkaline morning rituals not only nourishes your body but also establishes a positive mindset. Here's why these rituals matter:

1. **Hydration Kickstart:**

   o Begin your day with a glass of alkaline water. This helps rehydrate your body after a night's sleep and kickstarts your metabolism. Consider adding a splash of lemon for an extra alkaline boost.

2. **Mindful Preparation:**

   o Take a few moments to prepare your breakfast mindfully. Engage your senses in the process – the vibrant colors of fruits, the aroma of fresh ingredients, and the act of creating a nourishing meal. This sets a positive tone for the day ahead.

3. **Balanced Nutrition:**

   o Alkaline breakfasts provide a balanced mix of macronutrients and micronutrients. The combination of carbohydrates, proteins, and healthy fats ensures sustained energy levels throughout the morning, supporting both physical and mental activities.

4. **Digestive Harmony:**

- The alkaline-rich nature of these breakfasts supports a harmonious digestive environment. This can help prevent issues like bloating and indigestion, allowing you to move through your day with ease.

5. **Positive Intentions:**

   - Use your morning rituals as an opportunity to set positive intentions for the day. Reflect on what you're grateful for, visualize your goals, or simply embrace a moment of mindfulness. This mental preparation contributes to a more resilient and positive mindset.

CHAPTER 5

Lunches to Nourish and Sustain

Lunchtime – the midday refueling station for your body and mind. Chapter 5 is your guide to crafting lunches that not only nourish but also sustain, providing the energy and balance needed to power through the rest of your day. We'll explore alkaline lunch ideas suitable for both work and home, from vibrant salads and wraps to comforting warm dishes. Additionally, we'll delve into the art of balancing macronutrients in your alkaline meals, ensuring that every bite contributes to your overall well-being.

Alkaline Lunch Ideas for Work and Home

Whether you're packing lunch for the office or preparing a meal in the comfort of your home, these alkaline lunch ideas are both delicious and satisfying:

1. **Mediterranean Quinoa Salad:**
   - Ingredients: Cooked quinoa, cherry tomatoes, cucumber, olives, red onion, feta cheese, and a lemon vinaigrette.
   - Method: Toss the ingredients together, and you have a refreshing and nutrient-packed quinoa salad. It's a perfect balance of alkaline grains, colorful vegetables, and a touch of healthy fats from olives and feta.

2. **Chickpea and Avocado Wrap:**
   - Ingredients: Whole-grain wrap, mashed chickpeas, sliced avocado, shredded lettuce, and a drizzle of tahini dressing.
   - Method: Spread mashed chickpeas on a wrap, add sliced avocado and lettuce, then

drizzle with tahini dressing. This wrap is a portable powerhouse of plant-based protein and alkaline-rich ingredients.

3. **Warm Lentil Soup:**
   - Ingredients: Lentils, carrots, celery, onion, garlic, vegetable broth, and a dash of turmeric.
   - Method: Cook the lentils and vegetables in vegetable broth, season with turmeric, and you have a comforting warm lentil soup. It's a hearty and alkaline-rich option for a satisfying lunch.

4. **Quinoa and Vegetable Stir-Fry:**
   - Ingredients: Quinoa, broccoli, bell peppers, snap peas, tofu, and a soy-ginger sauce.
   - Method: Stir-fry the vegetables and tofu, add cooked quinoa, and toss with a soy-ginger sauce. This dish is a delightful combination of alkaline grains, colorful veggies, and plant-based protein.

5. **Spinach and Berry Salad with Almond Dressing:**

   o Ingredients: Fresh spinach, mixed berries, sliced almonds, and a dressing made with almond butter, lemon, and a touch of agave nectar.

   o Method: Toss the spinach and berries, sprinkle with sliced almonds, and drizzle with the almond dressing. This salad is a burst of flavors and textures that's as delicious as it is nutritious.

Salads, Wraps, and Warm Dishes

These lunch options go beyond mere sustenance; they are a symphony of flavors and textures that make every bite a delightful experience.

1. **Salads:**

   o Salads are not just a side dish; they can be the star of your lunch. Packed with fresh vegetables, leafy greens, and a variety of toppings, salads offer a canvas for creativity. The key is to include a mix of colors, textures, and nutrient-dense ingredients.

2. **Wraps:**

   o Wraps are a portable and versatile option. Whether it's a quinoa and vegetable wrap, a chickpea and avocado delight, or a Mediterranean-inspired creation, wraps provide a convenient way to enjoy a variety of alkaline-rich ingredients.

3. **Warm Dishes:**

   o Warm dishes add a comforting touch to your lunch. From lentil soup to quinoa stir-fry, these options provide a satisfying and nourishing meal that's perfect for colder days or when you crave something heartier.

Balancing Macronutrients in Alkaline Meals

The art of crafting an alkaline meal extends beyond choosing the right ingredients; it involves balancing macronutrients to support overall health. Let's break down the importance of balancing these components:

1. **Carbohydrates:**
   - Alkaline grains like quinoa and whole grains serve as excellent sources of complex carbohydrates. These provide a steady release of energy, helping to sustain you throughout the afternoon. Vegetables and fruits also contribute healthy carbohydrates, along with a myriad of essential vitamins and minerals.

2. **Proteins:**
   - Plant-based proteins are a cornerstone of alkaline meals. Whether it's the protein-packed chickpeas in a wrap, the tofu in a stir-fry, or the lentils in a warm soup, these sources of plant-based protein support muscle function, immune health, and overall vitality.

3. **Fats:**

o Healthy fats are essential for a well-rounded meal. Avocado, almonds, and olive oil are examples of sources that contribute monounsaturated and polyunsaturated fats. These fats support brain health, aid in nutrient absorption, and provide a sense of satiety.

4. **Fiber:**

   o Found abundantly in vegetables, fruits, and whole grains, fiber plays a crucial role in digestion and gut health. It adds bulk to your meals, contributing to a feeling of fullness and supporting a healthy digestive system.

5. **Micronutrients:**

   o In addition to macronutrients, alkaline meals are rich in micronutrients – vitamins and minerals that play vital roles in various bodily functions. The colorful array of fruits and vegetables in salads, wraps, and warm dishes ensures a diverse range of micronutrients that contribute to overall well-being.

Balancing these macronutrients ensures that your lunch is not only flavorful but also a comprehensive source of energy and nourishment.

CHAPTER 6

Dinners that Restore and Rejuvenate

As the day winds down, Chapter 6 invites you into the realm of dinners designed to restore and rejuvenate. These alkaline dinner recipes are crafted not only to nourish your body but also to usher in a peaceful night's rest. From the simplicity of grilled vegetables to the heartiness of alkaline grains and plant-based proteins, we'll explore the components that make these dinners a harmonious conclusion to your day. Additionally, we'll delve into mindful eating practices for the evening, guiding you towards a serene and balanced night.

Alkaline Dinner Recipes for a Peaceful Night's Rest

Dinner is more than just a meal; it's an opportunity to wind down, replenish, and prepare your body for a night of rejuvenating sleep. Let's explore some alkaline dinner recipes that align with this intention:

1. **Grilled Portobello Mushrooms with Quinoa:**
   - Ingredients: Portobello mushrooms, quinoa, cherry tomatoes, spinach, and balsamic glaze.
   - Method: Grill the portobello mushrooms and serve them over a bed of quinoa mixed with cherry tomatoes and spinach. Drizzle with balsamic glaze for a simple yet satisfying dinner rich in alkaline grains and vegetables.
2. **Lemon Herb Baked Salmon with Asparagus:**
   - Ingredients: Salmon fillet, asparagus, lemon, garlic, rosemary, and olive oil.
   - Method: Marinate the salmon with lemon, garlic, and rosemary, then bake it alongside asparagus. This dinner provides a dose of omega-3 fatty acids from the salmon and alkaline-rich asparagus.
3. **Chickpea and Vegetable Stir-Fry:**

- o Ingredients: Chickpeas, broccoli, bell peppers, snow peas, and a ginger-soy sauce.
- o Method: Stir-fry chickpeas and vegetables in a ginger-soy sauce for a quick and flavorful dinner. The chickpeas contribute plant-based protein, while the colorful veggies add alkaline goodness.

4. **Cauliflower and Chickpea Curry:**

- o Ingredients: Cauliflower, chickpeas, coconut milk, curry spices, and brown rice.
- o Method: Simmer cauliflower and chickpeas in a coconut milk-based curry sauce, and serve over brown rice. This dinner is a warm and comforting option that combines alkaline vegetables and grains.

5. **Zucchini Noodles with Pesto and Cherry Tomatoes:**

- o Ingredients: Zucchini noodles, homemade pesto, cherry tomatoes, and pine nuts.
- o Method: Toss zucchini noodles with pesto, cherry tomatoes, and pine nuts for a light

and refreshing dinner. Zucchini is an alkaline alternative to traditional pasta.

Grilled Vegetables, Alkaline Grains, and Plant-Based Proteins

The components of these dinners are carefully selected to create a synergy that not only satisfies your taste buds but also supports your body's need for restoration and rejuvenation.

1. **Grilled Vegetables:**
   - Grilled vegetables are a simple yet delightful addition to your dinner plate. Whether it's portobello mushrooms, asparagus, or a medley of colorful veggies, grilling enhances their natural flavors while preserving their nutritional integrity. The gentle cooking process retains the alkaline-rich goodness, making them a cornerstone of these dinners.

2. **Alkaline Grains:**

o Alkaline grains like quinoa and brown rice form the foundation of these dinners. These grains provide complex carbohydrates that are slowly released, offering sustained energy and supporting a peaceful transition into the night. The nutty flavor and versatile nature of these grains make them an excellent canvas for various dinner creations.

3. **Plant-Based Proteins:**

o Plant-based proteins, whether from chickpeas, lentils, or tofu, contribute to the nutritional completeness of these dinners. These proteins are not only alkaline-friendly but also offer a lighter alternative to animal proteins, making digestion smoother and contributing to a sense of balance.

4. **Healthy Fats:**

o Healthy fats from sources like olive oil, nuts, and avocados are incorporated to add richness to these dinners. These fats contribute to satiety, support nutrient absorption, and play a role in maintaining overall well-being.

Mindful Eating Practices for the Evening

As the evening sets in, adopting mindful eating practices can enhance your dinner experience and promote a sense of tranquility:

1. **Create a Calming Atmosphere:**
   - Set the tone for your evening meal by creating a serene environment. Dim the lights, play soft music, or light a candle to create a peaceful atmosphere that encourages mindful eating.
2. **Savor Each Bite:**
   - Take the time to savor each bite. Pay attention to the flavors, textures, and aromas of your dinner. This practice not only enhances your dining experience but also promotes better digestion.

3. **Chew Slowly:**

   o Chew your food slowly and thoroughly. This not only aids in digestion but also allows you to fully enjoy the taste and texture of your meal. It also sends signals to your brain that you are satisfied, preventing overeating.

4. **Put Away Screens:**

   o Create a screen-free zone during dinner. This means putting away smartphones, tablets, and TVs. Engage in conversation with family or simply enjoy the quietude of the evening.

5. **Express Gratitude:**

   o Take a moment to express gratitude for the nourishment your dinner provides. Reflect on the journey of the food from its source to your plate, cultivating an appreciation for the nourishing elements it brings to your body.

6. **Hydrate Mindfully:**

o While it's essential to stay hydrated, try to avoid excessive drinking during meals. Sipping water mindfully can enhance your dining experience without diluting digestive juices.

Adopting mindful eating practices transforms your dinner into a ritual of self-care, promoting relaxation and balance as you conclude your day.

CHAPTER 7

Snacks and Sweets for Guilt-Free Indulgence

Enter the realm of guilt-free indulgence with Chapter 7 – a treasure trove of alkaline snacks and sweets designed to satisfy your cravings without compromising on your commitment to a balanced lifestyle. This chapter is all about embracing the joy of nibbling between meals and relishing desserts that are not just delicious but also aligned with the principles of the alkaline diet. Let's explore the world of alkaline snack options, healthy dessert recipes, and how to seamlessly incorporate these treats into your daily life.

Alkaline Snack Options for Between Meals

Snacking doesn't have to be a guilty pleasure; it can be an opportunity to nourish your body between meals. Here are some alkaline snack options that are not only tasty but also support your well-being:

1. **Almond and Berry Parfait:**
   - Ingredients: Almonds, mixed berries, and coconut yogurt.
   - Method: Layer almonds, mixed berries, and coconut yogurt to create a parfait. This snack is a delightful blend of crunchy almonds, antioxidant-rich berries, and probiotic-packed coconut yogurt.
2. **Celery Sticks with Hummus:**
   - Ingredients: Celery sticks and homemade hummus.
   - Method: Dip celery sticks into homemade hummus for a refreshing and alkaline-rich

snack. Celery provides a satisfying crunch, while hummus adds protein and healthy fats.

3. **Cucumber and Avocado Slices:**
   - Ingredients: Cucumber slices and avocado.
   - Method: Top cucumber slices with avocado for a quick and hydrating snack. Avocado contributes healthy fats, while cucumber adds a dose of water and freshness.

4. **Chia Seed Pudding Cups:**
   - Ingredients: Chia seeds, almond milk, and a topping of sliced kiwi and strawberries.
   - Method: Mix chia seeds with almond milk, refrigerate until set, and top with sliced kiwi and strawberries. Chia seed pudding is a nutritious and satisfying snack that can also double as a dessert.

5. **Nuts and Dried Fruits Mix:**
   - Ingredients: Mixed nuts (almonds, walnuts, cashews) and dried fruits (apricots, figs).
   - Method: Create a personalized mix of your favorite nuts and dried fruits for a portable

and energizing snack. The combination of nuts and dried fruits provides a balance of healthy fats and natural sugars.

Healthy Dessert Recipes Without Compromising on Taste

Desserts can be a guilt-free pleasure with the right ingredients and a touch of creativity. Here are some healthy dessert recipes that allow you to indulge without compromising on taste:

1. **Berry and Almond Smoothie Bowl:**
   - Ingredients: Mixed berries, banana, almond milk, and a topping of sliced almonds.
   - Method: Blend mixed berries, banana, and almond milk into a smoothie, and top with sliced almonds. This dessert is not only visually appealing but also a refreshing and nutrient-packed treat.
2. **Coconut and Lime Energy Bites:**

- o Ingredients: Shredded coconut, dates, almonds, and lime zest.
- o Method: Blend shredded coconut, dates, almonds, and lime zest into a dough. Roll into bite-sized balls for a tropical-flavored energy boost. These bites are a guilt-free alternative to traditional sweets.

3. **Dark Chocolate-Dipped Strawberries:**
   - o Ingredients: Fresh strawberries and dark chocolate (70% cocoa or higher).
   - o Method: Melt dark chocolate and dip fresh strawberries for a decadent yet wholesome dessert. Dark chocolate is rich in antioxidants, and strawberries add a natural sweetness.

4. **Avocado Chocolate Mousse:**
   - o Ingredients: Ripe avocados, cocoa powder, maple syrup, and vanilla extract.
   - o Method: Blend avocados, cocoa powder, maple syrup, and vanilla extract into a silky chocolate mousse. This dessert is a creamy

and indulgent treat that sneaks in the health benefits of avocados.

5. **Baked Cinnamon Apples:**
   o Ingredients: Sliced apples, cinnamon, and a drizzle of honey.
   o Method: Toss sliced apples with cinnamon and bake until tender. Drizzle with honey for a warm and comforting dessert that captures the essence of apple pie without the guilt.

Incorporating Alkaline Treats into Your Lifestyle

The key to making alkaline treats a seamless part of your lifestyle is to approach them with balance and mindfulness. Here are some tips for incorporating these treats into your daily life:

1. **Portion Control:**
   o Enjoy treats in moderation. A small serving of a delicious snack or dessert can satisfy

your cravings without derailing your commitment to a balanced lifestyle.

2. **Intuitive Eating:**

   o Listen to your body's signals. Pay attention to hunger and fullness cues, and choose treats when you genuinely desire them rather than as a response to emotions or external cues.

3. **Homemade Goodness:**

   o Opt for homemade treats whenever possible. This gives you control over the ingredients, allowing you to create wholesome and satisfying options.

4. **Balanced Meals:**

   o Ensure that your main meals are balanced with alkaline-rich foods. This sets the foundation for incorporating treats without upsetting the overall alkaline balance in your diet.

5. **Mindful Enjoyment:**

o When you indulge in a treat, do so mindfully. Savor each bite, appreciate the flavors, and be present in the moment. This mindful approach enhances the enjoyment of the treat.

6. **Variety is Key:**

o Explore a variety of alkaline treats. This not only keeps your palate excited but also ensures that you are getting a diverse range of nutrients from different ingredients.

By adopting these principles, alkaline treats become a joyful addition to your lifestyle rather than a source of guilt or restriction.

CHAPTER 8

Beyond the Kitchen – Alkaline Living in Daily Life

Step into the final chapter of our alkaline journey, where we venture beyond the kitchen to explore how alkaline living extends into the fabric of daily life. Chapter 8 delves into the significance of alkaline hydration, the art of seamlessly incorporating alkaline habits into your daily routines, and a reflective exploration of the transformative journey to an alkaline lifestyle. This chapter serves as a guide to not only what you eat but how you live, inviting you to embrace a holistic approach to well-being.

Alkaline Hydration and the Importance of Water

Hydration is the cornerstone of well-being, and in the realm of alkaline living, the quality of water takes center stage. Let's understand the importance of alkaline hydration and how water can be a transformative element in your daily life.

1. **The pH Balance of Water:**
   - Alkaline water typically has a higher pH level than regular tap water, often ranging from 8 to 9.5. This higher pH is believed to help counteract the acidic load in the body, promoting a more balanced internal environment.

2. **Hydrating with Alkaline Water:**
   - Making alkaline water a part of your daily hydration routine is as simple as investing in a water filter or ionizer. This ensures that the water you consume aligns with the principles of the alkaline diet.

3. **Benefits of Alkaline Hydration:**

   o Advocates of alkaline water suggest that it may contribute to improved hydration, better absorption of nutrients, and enhanced detoxification. While scientific consensus on these claims is still evolving, staying well-hydrated with quality water remains a fundamental aspect of overall health.

4. **Balancing Acidic Foods:**

   o In the context of an alkaline diet, where certain foods may have an acidic impact on the body, alkaline water is seen by some as a counterbalance. It's like providing your body with a helping hand in maintaining equilibrium.

5. **Lemon-Infused Alkaline Water:**

   o Adding a slice of lemon to your alkaline water not only enhances the flavor but also contributes to alkalinity. Despite being acidic in nature, lemons have an alkalizing effect on the body once metabolized.

In essence, alkaline hydration is about making mindful choices regarding the water you consume, aiming for a pH balance that aligns with the principles of the alkaline lifestyle.

Incorporating Alkaline Habits into Daily Routines

Alkaline living isn't confined to the kitchen—it's a way of life that extends into your daily routines. Here's how you can seamlessly incorporate alkaline habits into various aspects of your day:

1. **Morning Rituals:**
   - Begin your day with a glass of alkaline water infused with lemon. This simple morning ritual not only hydrates your body but also kickstarts your metabolism and provides a gentle alkalizing effect.

2. **Mindful Movement:**
   - Incorporate mindful movement into your daily routine. This could be in the form of

yoga, stretching, or a leisurely walk. Movement supports circulation, digestion, and overall well-being.

3. **Alkaline Snacking:**

   o Keep alkaline snacks on hand for moments between meals. Whether it's a handful of nuts, sliced vegetables with hummus, or a piece of fruit, these snacks contribute to sustained energy and alkaline balance.

4. **Green Smoothie Breaks:**

   o Introduce green smoothie breaks into your day. A quick blend of alkaline greens, fruits, and water provides a nutrient boost that can be both refreshing and revitalizing.

5. **Hydrate Throughout the Day:**

   o Make a conscious effort to stay hydrated throughout the day. Set reminders to take water breaks, and consider having a reusable water bottle on hand to make hydration easily accessible.

6. **Mindful Meals:**

o Approach meals with mindfulness. Chew your food slowly, savoring each bite. This not only enhances the digestive process but also fosters a deeper connection with the act of nourishing your body.

7. **Evening Reflection:**

o Take a few moments in the evening for reflection. Consider aspects of your day that brought joy or presented challenges. This practice of self-awareness contributes to emotional well-being.

Incorporating alkaline habits into your daily life is about infusing intentionality into your routines, creating a tapestry of wellness that extends beyond individual meals.

Reflection on the Transformative Journey to an Alkaline Lifestyle

As you near the end of "The Alkaline Delight Cookbook," take a moment to reflect on the transformative journey to an alkaline lifestyle. Consider the following aspects:

1. **Awareness of Food Choices:**
   - Reflect on how your awareness of food choices has evolved. Have you become more attuned to the alkaline-forming nature of certain foods? How has this awareness influenced your culinary preferences?

2. **Nourishment and Vitality:**
   - Explore how the shift towards alkaline-rich foods has impacted your sense of nourishment and vitality. Have you noticed changes in energy levels, digestion, or overall well-being?

3. **Mindful Eating Practices:**
   - Consider the incorporation of mindful eating practices into your daily life. How has this mindful approach to meals influenced your relationship with food and your body?

4. **Holistic Well-Being:**

o Think about the holistic nature of alkaline living. Beyond the kitchen, how have alkaline habits touched other areas of your life, such as hydration, movement, and mindfulness?

5. **Challenges and Celebrations:**

o Acknowledge both challenges and celebrations along the way. Every journey has its ups and downs. What lessons have you learned from moments of difficulty, and how have you celebrated your successes?

6. **Sustainability of Habits:**

o Consider the sustainability of alkaline habits in your lifestyle. Which habits have seamlessly integrated into your daily routine, and how do they contribute to a sense of balance?

7. **Future Intentions:**

o Look ahead and set intentions for the future. How do you envision the continuation of an alkaline lifestyle? Are there areas you would like to explore further or refine in your journey?

Reflecting on your transformative journey to an alkaline lifestyle allows you to appreciate the progress made, learn from experiences, and set a positive trajectory for the future.

CONCLUSION

A Vibrant Life with The Alkaline Delight Cookbook

As we bring our culinary exploration to a close, let's reflect on the vibrant life that awaits you with The Alkaline Delight Cookbook. This journey has been a tapestry of flavors, a celebration of nourishing choices, and an invitation to embrace a holistic approach to well-being. In this conclusion, we'll recap the key principles and recipes that have guided you, offer encouragement to embrace a long-term alkaline lifestyle, and provide resources for further exploration and support on your continuing journey.

Recap of Key Principles and Recipes

1. **Alkaline Principles:**
    - The foundation of the alkaline lifestyle lies in the principles of balancing the body's pH, favoring alkaline-forming foods, and

minimizing acidic choices. This balance is believed to support overall health, vitality, and well-being.

2. **Key Alkaline Foods:**

   o Throughout The Alkaline Delight Cookbook, we've explored a variety of key alkaline foods. From vibrant fruits and vegetables to wholesome grains, plant-based proteins, and healthy fats, these ingredients form the palette for creating delicious and nourishing meals.

3. **Balancing Macronutrients:**

   o The art of balancing macronutrients—carbohydrates, proteins, and fats—has been a recurring theme. Each recipe is crafted not just for taste but with a mindful approach to supporting your body's need for sustained energy and overall nourishment.

4. **Mindful Eating Practices:**

   o Beyond the ingredients, we've delved into the importance of mindful eating practices.

From savoring each bite to adopting mindful mealtime rituals, these practices enhance the dining experience and promote a deeper connection with the food you consume.

5. **Holistic Living:**

   o The journey hasn't been confined to the kitchen. Alkaline living extends into daily routines, from morning rituals to mindful movement, hydration practices, and reflections on well-being. It's a holistic approach that transcends individual meals.

Encouragement to Embrace a Long-Term Alkaline Lifestyle

As you stand at the threshold of a vibrant life with The Alkaline Delight Cookbook, consider the following encouragement to embrace a long-term alkaline lifestyle:

1. **Celebrate Progress, Not Perfection:**

   o Embrace the journey with a spirit of celebration. Progress towards a more

alkaline lifestyle is a series of small steps
and mindful choices. Celebrate each positive
choice and acknowledge that perfection is
not the goal.

2. **Cultivate Mindful Awareness:**

    o   Cultivate mindful awareness in your
        relationship with food and your body. Listen
        to your body's signals, be present during
        meals, and approach eating as a joyful and
        nourishing experience.

3. **Find Joy in Exploration:**

    o   Alkaline living is a journey of exploration.
        Find joy in trying new recipes, discovering
        the flavors of alkaline-rich foods, and
        adapting your palate to a diverse range of
        nourishing ingredients.

4. **Connect with a Community:**

    o   Consider connecting with a community that
        shares similar wellness goals. Whether it's
        online forums, social media groups, or local
        gatherings, a supportive community can

provide encouragement, inspiration, and shared experiences.

5. **Adapt Recipes to Your Taste:**
    o The recipes in The Alkaline Delight Cookbook serve as a starting point. Feel free to adapt them to suit your taste preferences and dietary needs. The goal is to enjoy nourishing meals that resonate with your individual palate.

6. **Incorporate Alkaline Habits:**
    o Alkaline living goes beyond the plate. Incorporate alkaline habits into your daily life, from mindful hydration to movement and reflective moments. These habits contribute to a lifestyle that supports balance and vitality.

Resources for Further Exploration and Support

As you continue your journey, here are resources for further exploration and support:

1. **Alkaline Lifestyle Books:**

   o Explore additional books on the alkaline lifestyle for in-depth insights and inspiration. From cookbooks to guides on holistic well-being, there's a wealth of literature to deepen your understanding.

2. **Online Communities:**

   o Join online communities dedicated to the alkaline lifestyle. These communities provide a platform to share experiences, ask questions, and connect with individuals on similar journeys.

3. **Holistic Wellness Courses:**

   o Consider enrolling in holistic wellness courses that delve into the principles of alkaline living, mindfulness practices, and overall well-being. Online platforms offer a range of courses led by experts in the field.

4. **Nutritional Counseling:**

   o For personalized guidance, consider seeking the support of a nutritional counselor or holistic health practitioner. They can provide tailored advice based on your individual needs and wellness goals.

5. **Local Farmer's Markets:**

   o Explore local farmer's markets for a fresh and diverse selection of alkaline-friendly produce. Engaging with local farmers not only supports the community but also allows you to discover seasonal and nutrient-rich ingredients.

6. **Fitness and Wellness Events:**

   o Attend fitness and wellness events in your area. These events often feature workshops, cooking demonstrations, and opportunities to connect with like-minded individuals passionate about well-being.

In concluding your journey with The Alkaline Delight Cookbook, remember that it's not just about the recipes—it's about embracing a lifestyle that nurtures your body, mind, and spirit. Each choice, each mindful moment, contributes to the vibrant life you're creating. As you continue forward, may your days be filled with the delight of nourishing foods, the joy of mindful living, and the energy of holistic well-being. Here's to the vibrant life you deserve!